BIG BOLD AND BEAUTIFUL

Loving yourself regardless of your body size

Theresa Lovic

TABLE OF CONTENTS

CHAPTER 1

A bitter truth

These days the media is assaulting us with their image of what the ideal physique should look like. We're treated to these pictures as tiny girls and see them every single day. In periodicals, in advertising, on television… there is virtually no escape from it all.

This is why I'm liking this entire "Body Positivity" trend that is going around at the moment.

As someone who sees herself as plus size, it's been challenging. I dread shopping since the majority of businesses on the high street exclusively cater to ladies of a smaller size. I've had people criticize me for eating an extra piece of pizza and even had others send me "gifts" of stuff to help me lose weight.

Now, don't get me wrong, I DO want to lose weight, and I DO want to be healthy. There are days I'd give my right arm to be able to fit into a size ten pair of trousers or not have my parts wobble when I run. What I'm saying is, that I'm not going to allow the fact I'm larger to hold me back in life. All too often I hear my smaller friends tell me that they won't allow themselves to purchase any new clothing until they're lowered two dress sizes, or no snacks until they've lost 5lbs and you know what? That makes me incredibly sad. As much as I'd want to be smaller, why should anybody have to put their life on hold until they're at their ideal weight? Where does it end? If you lose all that weight, are you still going to be happy? Is it going to miraculously make your life perfect? Probably not. People could treat you better, and you may have more confidence for a brief time but if those concerns you have about your physique and self-worth are so deep based then you have to focus on yourself first.

Each year, the dieting industry is earning millions off of our fears. Offering their magic weight reduction solution that would help you alter your life. Sure, you'll be unhappy as hell for a few months but you'll look fantastic in a bikini (for a week or two)… then if you go back to normal you'll gain all that weight and thus the vicious cycle begins again. All while these folks who are selling you their magical weight reduction solution are laughing all the way to the bank.

If working out at the gym for 10 hours a week and eating nothing but veggies is your thing then that is fantastic and I salute you. But for me, I find joy in eating nice meals. I like to indulge in a cake and a foamy cappuccino every once in a while. I'm not suggesting "let us all sit on our arses and eat crap" — far from it. Eating well and exercising are extremely crucial for your health. What I am saying is that life is much too short to be miserable in your flesh. Don't deny yourself just so society can accept you. If you want to appear attractive, go within yourself and concentrate on that first. Then go out, and purchase that new outfit you've been eyeing. Go get your hair trimmed and fresh lippy. Go to the beach with your kids and wear a bikini. Don't wait to be tiny before you can enjoy your life. Enjoy yourself. The sexiest thing about a lady is confidence.

Regardless of your size, as women (including guys) we all have anxieties. You see some of the ladies around and behind closed doors, they're secretly dissatisfied because their boobs aren't large enough/too big or they dislike their legs or their arms, etc.

Nobody is perfect... and it in itself is great. We are all born to be different. We're all of various shapes and sizes. That in itself is wonderful.

So your task for today is to think up three things you appreciate about your body. There has to be something. Leave a comment with three things you love about your body, I'd love to know.

Do something every day that makes you feel good about yourself. Dress up, look in the mirror and tell yourself that you're beautiful. And don't let the way you look hold you back from enjoying life.

CHAPTER 2

How To Love Your Body: 10 Small Ways To Start, Even When It's Hard

Maybe you despise your body. Or maybe you simply wish your physique looked different. You're not alone: Research shows up to 84% of American women feel body dissatisfaction throughout their lives. Learning to love your body when you don't is no easy process, and it's not as straightforward as the body positivity movement may sometimes make it appear. Going from "I detest my body" to something more positive will require time and intentional effort. Here are a few modest, real methods to start:

1. Commit to it

"The fact that you realize you want to change is how you start to change. Congratulations. Acknowledgment is 50% of the effort."

The first step to altering how you feel about your body is committing to the change. You need to accept that you have a poor connection with your body and that you want to have a good, healthy one. Tell yourself, I want to have a good connection with my body, and make sure you mean it!

2. Ditch the narrative that looking a certain way will make you happier.

Ask yourself this: Why do you want to look different?

Most likely, it's because you want other people to like you, and you believe looking a certain way will make you more loved and accepted.

"We are sold this idea that looking a certain way will bring us approval, affection, love, respect, value, etc.

Before you can learn to love your body, you need to relinquish the idea that you wouldn't feel sad, lonely, or rejected if you looked different. "

Even Beyoncé got cheated on! Human life involves beauty and suffering for everyone,".

"The more you have this idea, the less attached you will be to meeting certain conventional beauty norms because you will understand that they will never deliver what you want. Peace and happiness have to come from inside."

This isn't to say that size discrimination, racism, and ableism aren't real—yes, unfortunately, these physical factors do affect how people treat us. But bending over backward to meet their impossible ideals will not help you feel better about yourself. Is your body the problem, or are ideals the problem? Instead of continuing to try to fit into a system that pits you against your own body, what if you adopted a new way of thinking that designates you as valuable exactly the way you are? What if you stopped trying to appease others at your own expense?

Try repeating this to yourself: I deserve to be loved and accepted in this exact body. I will no longer entertain persons or communications that tell me differently.

3. Cleanse your social media feeds of everything that makes you feel horrible about your body.

Those super skinny glamorous-looking celebs and reality TV competitors you follow on Instagram? You may believe they're innocuous to scroll past, but study tells us time and time again that exposure to media showcasing unrealistic body types is linked to poor body image. Take control of what images and messages you allow into your brain. Look at the accounts you are following. Do they make you feel empowered? Delete and add new accounts as necessary because what you surround yourself with influences you, no matter how immune you may think you are to those images."

4. Get to know your body.

To love your body, you must first know your body.

"The body is the physical manifestation of emotions, and this has nothing to do with how it appears or how old it is,". Once you are acquainted with your body's language (not body language), you are better equipped to recognize what it's attempting to tell you. Slowing down to heed your body's signals is how you build compassion—which is a sort of love.

There are so many methods to get to know your body on a deeper level. For example, if you've got a uterus, consider documenting your menstrual cycle in greater detail. Consider trying something like a menstrual cup to manage your periods, as the act of inserting and removing a cup forces you to feel out your cervix with your fingers, see and feel your monthly blood, and overall become personal with your body. Or you can consider attempting a sort of exercise or movement that demands a lot of control of the body—belly dance, weightlifting, or even yoga. You'd be shocked how much getting to know your body better can make it so much easier to love.

5. *Do something that makes your body feel wonderful everyday.*

Make it a habit to do something nice for your body every day. Maybe that's setting out a few minutes to simply give yourself a hand massage. Maybe it's putting on your softest, fuzziest pair of socks to wear about the home. Maybe it's applying a rejuvenating face mask or putting on a full face of makeup for no reason other than it makes you feel wonderful.

This is all about educating your brain to correlate your body with good thoughts. Make it a practice to shower your body with affection, and it'll start to seem natural and intuitive over time.

6. Feed your senses.

"Any time that I am feeling any sort of way about my body, I'm typically removed from it and I'm usually disconnected from the joyful experience of having a body—of being able to taste tasty foods, to view beautiful sights, to hear things," Whitney adds. "Our bodies are geared for pleasure. The entire point of having a body is for us to feel good."

Feed your senses, she suggests. Interact with them. "That builds body connection, and that body connection helps dismantle the body hatred.

7. Practice appreciation for your body.

"It's so much more useful to think about what our bodies do for us daily, "Our bodies carry us through our days with so much power and elegance. Our bodies are also capable of unlimited levels of pleasure! If we can be appreciative for all the things our bodies do for us, it might help us view them from a new perspective."

8. Make exercise about feeling good.

"When it comes to exercise, it is wonderful to have people define it as moving your body in a manner that makes you joyful. Exercise in a manner that provides you delight,". "We want to frame this as a means to appreciate our body, not beat it down until it's into a form that pleases us."

An exercise is a natural approach to enhancing energy, decreasing stress, and keeping our bodies healthy. But when we look at exercise as a weight reduction or body-shaping technique, we convert something healthy into something painful and even cruel to our bodies. Exercise as a method to embrace your body—not as a way to alter or resist it.

9. Dress your body gently.

Sometimes when we're feeling uncomfortable about our bodies, we intentionally or unconsciously put on clothing aimed to cover up as much of our body's "problem areas" as possible or draw the least amount of attention. This bolsters shame and negativity surrounding our bodies.

 Dress your body like it's a piece of artwork. Be deliberate, attentive, and expressive. If you're financially able, treat yourself to a shopping trip and purchase clothing that makes you feel good and makes your body feel wonderful. When we clothe our body purposefully, we're treating it as something deserving of care and affection. We give the message—to others and ourselves—that this is a body that is loved.

10. Do mirror work.

Learning to embrace your body will not happen suddenly. Small daily routines are crucial to going ahead on this road and progressively educating your mind over time to cease being so judgemental of your body. One wonderful habit is a positive affirmation exercise done in front of a mirror: Take a minute each morning to look at your complete body and say something positive about it. You can also wish to specify the regions of your body that you don't like to concentrate your positive affirmations on. For example, if you detest your thighs, you may try chanting to yourself: I adore my big thighs, or My thighs are powerful and seductive.

Importantly, though, don't push love if it's not there just yet. "

If you don't get there, it will be another cause to beat yourself up. Stop adding on the humiliation. That may be too much, too extreme, or darn near impossible for you at this moment in your progress. Can you try to uncover a few items that you possibly appreciate instead? Maybe you have wonderful hands, or ankles, or gorgeous eyes, fantastic shoulders, or amazing hair."

CHAPTER 3

Admiring your body

So frequently we take our body for granted. All too often we mistreat our body with our inattention or self-critical comments: "You are too overweight. You are too slim. You aren't attractive enough. You aren't quick enough. You aren't athletic enough. Your chin is too pointed. Your hips are excessively broad. You are too hairy." The body hears all these criticisms and continues to work dutifully. What patient bodies we have absorbed so much neglect and hatred!

Consider how much of your thought time you dedicate to self-criticism. Let's be genuine here. Have you noticed yourself changing your shirt or jeans because you don't like the way you appear in your clothes? Do you feel awful about eating food because you believe your physique is too big? As you connect with someone of the other sex, are you self-conscious, wondering whether they would be attracted to a physique that you deem "just not good enough"? Isn't it odd that we detest our looks and believe we don't measure up?"

Each of us is trying to strut our things and dress ourselves up so we appear beautiful yet below the stylish clothes and cosmetics, we ALL feel "less than" the others. Even the models in the publications worry their bodies aren't good enough. If gorgeous individuals don't feel pretty, then how can anyone? I suppose that the Eternal Source must look down on us with compassion observing the needless pain that comes with our unhappiness.

It's time for every one of us to wake up and understand that we have amazing bodies!

What do we utilize our bodies for? They help us to navigate and appreciate the world around us. Through our bodies, we encounter lovely smells and harsh aromas. We feel the tenderness of a child's touch and the thorns of a cactus. We notice the many blues of the sky and the greens and browns of the terrain. We relish sweet plantains and flavorful fish stew. We delight at the sight of our loved ones and embrace them with hugs and good words.

 What incredible things our bodies are allowing us to experience with very little awareness on our part!

Take a fresh look at your physique. First, look into your own eyes and sense your eternal spirit. This is the True You. Your spirit is utilizing this body to experience life on Earth. For a minute put aside your reservations about your looks.

Instead, look at the remarkable traits your body is endowed with. Every aspect is meaningful and all are properly connected.

Finally, consider the opinion of Queen Latifah, "For me, it may seem cliché, but beauty for me truly does originate on the inside. It's like a state of mind, a state of love if you will. Then, everything you can accomplish on the outside is all like a bonus."